GASTRIC SLEEVE COOKBOOK

Top 50 Delicious Mexican Cuisine Recipes

ROSIE CARRIER

© Copyright 2018 by Rosie Carrier - All rights reserved.

The following book is reproduced below with the goal of providing information that is as accurate and reliable as possible. Regardless, purchasing this book can be seen as consent to the fact that both the publisher and the author of this book are in no way experts on the topics discussed within and that any recommendations or suggestions that are made herein are for entertainment purposes only. Professionals should be consulted as needed prior to undertaking any of the action endorsed herein.

This declaration is deemed fair and valid by both the American Bar Association and the Committee of Publishers Association and is legally binding throughout the United States.

Furthermore, the transmission, duplication or reproduction of any of the following work including specific information will be considered an illegal act irrespective of if it is done electronically or in print. This extends to creating a secondary or tertiary copy of the work or a recorded copy and is only allowed with an expressed written consent from the Publisher. All additional rights reserved.

The information in the following pages is broadly considered to be truthful and accurate account of facts, and as such any inattention, use or misuse of the information in question by the reader will render any resulting actions solely under their purview. There are no scenarios in which the publisher or the original author of this work can be in any fashion deemed liable for any hardship or damages that may befall them after undertaking information described herein.

Additionally, the information in the following pages is intended only for informational purposes and should thus be thought of as universal. As befitting its nature, it is presented without assurance regarding its prolonged validity or interim quality. Trademarks that are mentioned are done without written consent and can in no way be considered an endorsement from the trademark holder.

TABLE OF CONTENTS

Introduction 1
    Pre-Surgery Meals 1
    Post-Op Diet 4
    Picking Appropriate Foods 7
    Complications 8

Beef and Pork 10
    Taco Stew (Dairy Free) 10
    Steak Fajitas (Dairy Free) 12
    Taco Pie (Low Carb) 14
    Slow Cooker Carnitas "Nachos" (Low Carb) 15
    Bacon Sliders (Low Carb) 17
    Taco Beef (Low Carb, Dairy Free) 19
    Chipotle Steak Salad (Low Carb) 21
    Chile Relleno Casserole (Low Carb) 22
    Steak and Mushroom Fajita Sandwiches 23
    Pork and Black Bean Stew (Dairy Free) 25

Poultry 27
    Chicken Skillet 27
    Salsa Verde Stuffed Poblanos (Low Carb, Dairy Free) 28
    Taco Casserole (Low Carb) 30
    Chili Lime Jalapeno Turkey Burgers (Low Carb, Dairy Free) 31
    Cilantro Lime Chicken with Tomato Relish (Low Carb, Dairy Free) 33

Turkey Skillet with Salsa and Eggs (Low Carb, Dairy Free) 35

Chicken Chili with Jalapeno and Cheddar (Low Carb) 36

Soft Mexican Chicken Salad (Low Carb, Dairy Free) 37

Grilled Chicken with Pico de Gallo (Low Carb, Dairy Free) 38

Turkey Taco Meatballs (Low Carb) 40

Slow cooker Salsa Chicken (Low Carb) 41

Slow Cooker Chicken Fajitas 42

Slow cooker Tex Mex Chicken (Dairy Free) 44

Spinach and Chicken Flautas 45

Slow cooker Chicken Enchiladas 48

Creamy Green Chile Enchilada Soup 50

Chicken Avocado Casserole (Low Carb) 53

Seafood 55

Spicy Shrimp Burrito Bowl (Dairy Free) 55

Shrimp Tacos (Dairy Free) 58

Chipotle and Garlic Shrimp (Dairy Free, Low Carb) 60

Salmon with Mexican Rice Salad (Dairy Free) 61

Pacific Cod with Fajita Vegetables (Dairy Free) 63

Lemon Garlic Shrimp (Dairy Free) 65

Tilapia Veracruz (Dairy Free, Low Carb) 67

Salmon with Summer Salsa (Dairy Free) 69

Vegetables 70

Cilantro Lime Cauliflower Rice (Dairy Free, Low Carb) 70

Sweet Pepper Poppers (Low Carb) 71

Roasted Corn Guacamole 73

Bean and Spinach Burrito 75

Stuffed Southwest Style Sweet Potatoes (Dairy Free) 77

Vegetable Chili (Dairy Free) 79

Corn and Black Bean Salad (Dairy Free).......................................81

Spicy Peanut Vegetarian Chili (Dairy Free) 82

Black Bean, Rice, and Zucchini Skillet 84

Seven Layer Mexican Salad 86

Soft Foods 89

Scrambled Eggs with Black Bean Puree 89

Black Bean and Lime Puree 91

Pureed Salsa and Beans 92

Egg-Chillida (Low Carb) 93

Fat-Free Polenta 94

Conclusion 95

Introduction

Congratulations on purchasing *Gastric Sleeve Cookbook* and thank you for doing so.

Gastric sleeve surgery is a big step on the road to a healthy lifestyle, and it is one that shouldn't be taken lightly. These types of surgeries are typically the last option that a doctor will turn to, but they are extremely effective ways to lose weight when other methods have failed.

While making the decision to undergo this type of surgery is between you and your doctor, it helps to be prepared before the surgery. Knowing what you can and can't cook will help to take some of the stress out of the situation.

Right before the surgery, you will be put on a strict liquid diet. After the surgery, you will go through a step down from liquid to solid foods. But that doesn't mean that you can't enjoy what you consume.

This book is here to help take some of the stress away from this process. You will find 50 different Mexican recipes that you can enjoy at different stages in your healing process. There are even soft food Mexican recipes that you can enjoy shortly after your surgery.

The great thing is, you can also enjoy these before your surgery, at least before you go on the liquid diet. Just because you are limited on foods you can eat doesn't mean that you have to sacrifice flavor.

All of these recipes are high in protein so that you stay fuller longer. You will also find the serving size so that you know exactly how many people you can share with and know how much you should eat.

Pre-Surgery Meals

A gastric sleeve surgery is often used as a lifesaving procedure. You are going to lose weight and you will reduce your co-morbidities. After the surgery, you will find that you feel and look better. However, in order for the surgery to be a complete success, you will have to change your diet for the long term.

This may sound simple, but it really isn't. There will be a struggle. You have spent the majority of your life reinforcing and building up your bad eating habits, but all of those have to change, and pretty much instantly after the surgery. Otherwise, bad and painful things can end up happening.

Knowing the things that you can and can't eat is the best first step when it comes to eating a healthy diet. The diet that you consume during the first five weeks after you undergo gastric sleeve surgery is important for two reasons:

1. Your health and safety. Eating the wrong types of food could end up putting undue pressure on your stomach, which will still be healing.
2. Resetting and replacing your bad eating habits with new habits that will keep you healthy and happy.

To help reduce the amount of fat that is located around your spleen and liver, you will be put on a preoperative liquid diet. It will have to be followed for 7 to 14 days prior to your gastric sleeve surgery. If you do not follow this liquid diet correctly, then the surgery may be cancelled or delayed intra-operatively. This means that if they start the surgery and find that there is still a lot of fat around your spleen and liver, they will stop the procedure.

I really can't stress enough how important it will be for you to follow the pre-op liquid fast to the tee. You have probably been waiting 6 months to a year to get the go ahead for the surgery. Make sure you follow what the doctor tells you to do.

If you have an enlarged liver, it will prevent your surgeon from being able to see certain parts during the procedure. When the liver is too large, things become unsafe when performing a gastric sleeve surgery. This pre-op diet will typically involve the following elements:

- Meal replacement shakes or protein shakes will be the main components of your diet.
- You can only consume sugar-free beverages during this time. You can use sugar substitutes like Stevia.
- You cannot have carbonated or caffeinated beverages.
- You can have soup broth without any solid pieces of food.
- Vegetable juices and V8 are allowed.
- You can consume extremely thin cream of rice or cream of wheat.
- One to two daily servings of lean meat and vegetables could be okay, but this is only if you have them approved by a license healthcare professional

You have to make sure that you sip your liquids and beverages very slowly. You should not consume any types of beverages when you are consuming your meals, and you should wait at least 30 minutes after you have eaten a meal before you consume any type of liquid.

The purpose of this fast is to put your body into ketosis. This will let you body use up its fat stores as a form of energy. This will result in the fat from your liver shrinking considerably in a very short amount of time. Some of the best options for your high protein meal replacement shakes are:

- GNC Total Lean Shake 25
- Chike
- Unjury

- Isopure
- EAS Myoplex Light/Carb Control
- Bariatric Advantage

Post-Op Diet

After you have undergone your gastric sleeve surgery, you will be placed on a strict post operative diet plan that you will have to follow. Part of your stomach has been removed and you have to make sure that it is given the proper amount of time to heal. There are certain types of foods that can disrupt this healing process. If you put undue stress on the staples in your stomach, you can end up developing a leak.

There are four stages to this diet.

Week one you will consume clear liquids only. This means for the seven days following your surgery, you can only consume clear liquids; about one to two oz. per hour. Your dietitian will decide how long you need to stay in this phase, and they will suggest all the necessary guidelines you should follow. When it comes to the types of liquids you can have, these include:

- Sugar-free gelatin
- Fat- free broth
- Fat-free milk
- Water

During weeks two to three, you will move to protein shakes and pureed foods. This stage, most of the time, will only last for one week, but will sometimes last for two.

Since you now have a smaller stomach size, you will want to eat several smaller meals during your day. You need to have a daily intake of about 60 to 70 grams of protein. The protein can come from pureed fish, meat, egg whites, and protein shakes. You should also have around 64 oz. of clear liquids. This does not include the fluids from the pureed foods.

You should still stay away from carbonated and caffeinated beverages. You need to also say away from simple carbohydrates and sugar, as well as sugar alcohols. All of your foods should be pureed with fat-free broth, fat-free milk, or water. You should not consume clear liquids at the same time as you eat your pureed foods. As a guideline, you should not consume any clear liquids 30 minutes before and 60 minutes after a meal. You have to sip your clear liquids extremely slowly, and you should never use straws because they could end up bringing unwanted air into your stomach.

To make sure that you don't have any nutrient deficiencies, you can take one or two multivitamins that contain iron each day. You need to make sure that your multivitamins are in chewable or liquid form.

During weeks four and five, you get to move to soft foods. This is when you can slowly start to add in soft foods and it will typically last one to two weeks. If a food is able to be easily mashed with a spoon, fork, or knife, then you can consume it during this stage. You can eat soft meats as well as cooked vegetables. You should aim for 60 to 70 grams of protein and consume 64 oz. of fluids. You will likely consume three to six small meals each day.

During the last stage, you get to eat solid foods again. Now you can eat real food. Your diet should consist of protein, vegetables, a small amount of grains, and very few refined sugars. This is how you should try to eat for the rest of your life as well.

The best thing to do is to:

- Introduce a single new food at a time. Ideally, it would be no more than a single new food a day so that you are able to gauge how your body will react.

- Make sure you eat slowly. Chew your food extremely thoroughly, 15 seconds per bit. You can even get the Baritastic app, which will time your chewing.

- Make sure you separate your food and water by at least 30 minutes.

- Make sure that you consume at least 64 oz. of water each day.

- Make sure to eat your protein first, veggies second, and carbs third. Ideally, your carbs should be healthy grains or fruits, and not processed.

- Eat foods that are real and nutrient dense. Try to stay away from processed and pre-packaged foods that have a lot of ingredients.

- Read all nutrient labels. Try to focus on foods that are low in carbohydrates, and that have a calorie to protein ratio of ten to one or less. To do this, add a zero to the grams of proteins and if the total number of calories still comes out to more than that, then you should probably avoid that food, especially if you are having problems reaching your protein goals.

Once you are back on solid foods, all of the guidelines from stage three should still be followed. You dietician will probably give you a list of supplements that you should take to make sure that your body gets all the nutrients that it needs. You can also start to consume more vegetables and fruits, both raw and cooked. You can eat small amounts of fat, and extremely small amounts of sugar. You can also consume caffeinated and carbonated beverages in small amounts.

Your total caloric intake each day should be somewhere between 800 to 1200 and all the way up to 1500 18 months after your surgery.

In stage two you will also have been instructed to start physical activity. Hiking, badminton, canoeing, aerobics, weight lifting, biking, running, walking, and dancing around your bedroom like a crazy person are all great things that you can add to your weekly routine. Make sure that you try to aim for 30 minutes of exercise five to seven days each week. It doesn't matter *what* you do, it just matters *that* you do.

Make sure that you don't pick up anything that weights more than 10 lbs. for the first six weeks after your surgery. This could end up harming your internal stitches and cause a hernia.

Picking Appropriate Foods

When you are picking out foods to eat, you will want to go with choices that are high to moderate protein, low in carbs, and moderate in healthy fats. Foods that are high in healthy fats are:

- Coconut oil
- Nut butter
- Sardines
- Nuts
- Salmon
- Avocados

A general guideline for picking foods is:

- Pick very lean meats.
- Canned salmon and tuna.
- Stay away from spicy and greasy foods. You can introduce spice later on in moderation.
- Stay away from whole milk.

- Consume foods that are nutrient dense; eggs, meats, veggies, and fruits.
- Plan out your meals.
- Make sure your family stays involved in your healthy eating choices.
- Shop for healthy foods.
- Try to limit or completely eliminate desserts.
- Keep temptations at bay by getting rid of junk foods.
- Cut out fast food.
- Eat out on occasion.
- Make sure you take quality nutritional vitamins and supplements.
- Keep your food and water separated by at least 30 minutes.
- Introduce all new foods slowly.
- Your meals should not be any larger than your fist.

Complications

Dumping syndrome is the most common complication that you may experience after your surgery, especially once you start eating solid foods. Dumping syndrome will happen when sweet or fatty foods are consumed too quickly or in too large of an amount.

When this happens, the stomach will dump the food into the small intestine before the stomach has had time to properly break it down. When dumping syndrome occurs you will likely feel nauseous, have cramps, diarrhea, vomiting, sweating, or an increase in your heart rate. These symptoms will typically go away after an hour or two. However, dumping syndrome is very unpleasant, so it is best that you do what you can to avoid this from happening.

To help you reduce the risk of experiencing dumping syndrome, you should:

- Chew your food completely.
- Eat in a slow and steady manner.
- Avoid consuming refined carbohydrates or high sugar foods.

You will find that there are certain foods that are more difficult to digest than others and you should consume them with caution:

- Beans
- Corn
- Whole grains
- Nuts
- Grapes
- Shellfish
- Pork
- Beef

No matter what type of meal you're looking for, beef, pork, veggie, chicken, or seafood, there is something in here for you. I'd even bet that your family will enjoy these recipes. Getting healthy and staying healthy doesn't have to be boring. With some spices and creativity, you can have a delicious healthy meal. Don't wait; start trying all of these delicious recipes today.

Beef and Pork

Taco Stew (Dairy Free)

4 – servings

What You Need:

1. Sliced green onions, .25 c
2. Undrained diced tomatoes and green chilis, 10 oz. can
3. Diced red bell pepper
4. Diced carrot, 1 c
5. Minced dried garlic, .5 tsp.
6. Low sodium taco seasoning, 1 packet
7. 93% lean ground beef, 1 lb.

What You Do:

1. Place a skillet on the stove and heat to medium high. Add in the ground beef and allow it to cook until it is completely browned. Break the beef apart as it cooks. Drain off any fat that has accumulated.
2. Mix the minced garlic and the taco seasoning packet into the cooked ground beef. Stir everything together until well combined and then allow it to cook and heat for two minutes. Add this meat into the bottom of your slow cooker.
3. Into your slow cooker, and on top of the beef, add in the canned tomatoes and green chilis, red bell pepper and carrots. Place the

lid on your cooker and then set it to low and allow it to cook for four to six hours.

4. Scoop the stew out and top it with the green onions. This recipe can easily be cooked on the stove top as well if you don't have a slow cooker. All you have to do is cook the ground beef and mix in the seasonings and add the results to a Dutch oven. Mix in all the other ingredients and let it cook until the carrots have softened.

Steak Fajitas (Dairy Free)

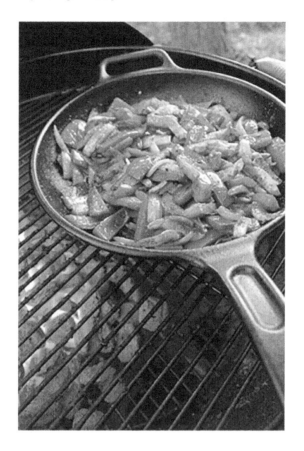

4 – servings

What You Need:

1. Salsa
2. Onion that has been sliced into strips
3. Green bell pepper that has been sliced into strips
4. Dried thyme, .5 tsp.
5. Mustard powder, .5 tsp.
6. Black pepper, 1 tsp.
7. Cumin, 1 tsp.

8. Dried rosemary, 2 tsp.
9. Chili powder, 2 tsp.
10. Natural sweetener, 2 packets
11. Paprika, 1 T
12. Sea salt, 1 T
13. Lean sirloin steak, 1 lb., cut into strips

What You Do:

1. Place all of the salt, paprika, sweetener, chili powder, dried rosemary, cumin, pepper, mustard powder, and dried thyme into a bowl and mix well to combine. Take out one tsp. of this mixture and reserve. Rub the steak slices really well with the spice mixture that you just made. Cover the steak and allow it to marinate until you are ready to cook it.

2. Place a large skillet on the stove and heat to medium high. Add the onion and pepper to the skillet along with spice mixture that you set to the side earlier. You need to cook the onion and peppers until they have softened up and the onions turn translucent. Take off heat and place in a bowl. Cover to keep warm.

3. Into the same skillet, add half the seasoned steak and cook about two minutes per side or until done to your liking. Place cooked steak onto a clean plate and cover until the rest of the steak gets done.

4. Once all the steak strips are done, add everything back into the skillet and warm everything up for a few minutes. Spoon onto plates and enjoy.

Taco Pie (Low Carb)

8 – servings

What You Need:
1. 2% cheddar cheese, .66 c, shredded
2. Pepper
3. Salt
4. Large eggs, 6
5. Water, .75 c
6. Taco seasoning packet
7. 93% lean ground beef, 1 lb.
8. Toppings of choice

What You Do:
1. Start out by placing your oven on 350.
2. Place a large skillet on stove top and heat to medium high. Once the skillet has heated up, add the ground beef and cook about five minutes breaking it apart as it cooks. Cook it until it is completely browned and no longer pink. If there is any fat, drain it off. Add water and taco seasoning packet. Stir well and simmer until water has been absorbed about 5 minutes.
3. Spray a 9-inch pie pan with cooking spray. Spread the beef mixture into the pie pan evenly.
4. Crack the eggs into a large bowl and season with pepper and salt. Whisk until well combined. Pour eggs over beef mixture and tilt the pie pan to make sure eggs cover the beef mixture completely.
5. Sprinkle cheese on top. Place in preheated oven and bake for about 25 minutes. After 25 minutes check pie and see if the eggs are set. If not, cook an additional 5 minutes. When done, take out of the oven and allow it to cool. Slice evenly and serve with toppings of choice.

Slow Cooker Carnitas "Nachos" (Low Carb)

6 – servings

What You Need:

1. Mini sweet peppers, 1 bag
2. Salt, .75 tsp.
3. Cumin, 1 T
4. Chicken broth, 10 oz. can
5. Chipotle peppers in adobo sauce, 7 oz. can
6. Minced garlic, 4 cloves
7. Lean pork shoulder, 2 lbs.

Toppings:

1. Cilantro, chopped, 2 T
2. 2% shredded cheddar cheese, .5 c

What You Do:

3. If you don't like cleaning a slow cooker, use a slow cooker liner or spray it well with some cooking spray. Place the chicken broth, chipotle peppers along with the sauce, salt, cumin, and garlic in the bottom of the slow cooker. Stir well to combine. Add the pork shoulder and turn to coat all sides.
4. Place the pork shoulder in your slow cooker and sit the lid on top. Turn the slow cooker onto low and set for six hours. When done, take the pork out of slow cooker and shred using two forks. Place back into slow cooker and stir to coat pork with sauce.
5. Warm your oven to 350. Cut the bell pepper in half and take out seeds and ribs. Place evenly onto a baking pan. Spread

shredded pork onto bell peppers evenly. Sprinkle with cheese. Place in preheated oven and bake for 10 minutes.

6. Once the cheese is melted, take out of oven and top with toppings of choice. Enjoy.

Bacon Sliders (Low Carb)

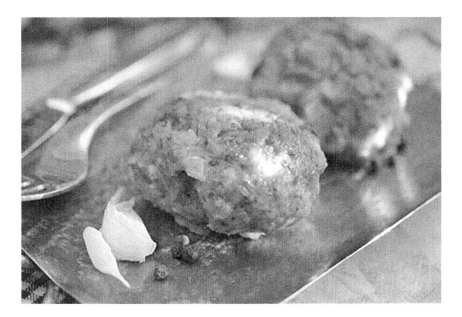

6 – servings

What You Need:

1. Reduced fat cheddar cheese, 3 oz., cut into six cubes
2. Diced tomatoes with green chilies, 1 c, divided, undrained
3. Onion powder, .5 tsp
4. Turkey bacon, cooked and crumbled, 4 slices
5. Fresh spinach, 1 c tightly packed and chopped
6. 93 % lean ground beef, 1 lb.

What You Do:

1. The first thing that you need to do is grease up your grill, and then allow it to heat to medium high.
2. Add two T of tomatoes, and all of the onion powder, bacon, spinach, and ground beef to a bowl and mix well to combine. Divide into 6 parts and shape into meatballs.

3. Take each cheese cube and put one into the center of each meatball. Make sure the cheese is completely covered with meat. Flatten to make into a burger shape.

4. Place onto heated grill and cook for 5 minutes. Flip and cook another 5minutes until done to your likeness. Make sure the center reaches 160 degrees to kill off any bacteria.

5. Take off heat and place onto plates. Top with remaining tomatoes. Enjoy.

Taco Beef (Low Carb, Dairy Free)

6 – servings

What You Need:

1. Chipotle pepper in adobo sauce, minced, just 1
2. Minced garlic, 5 cloves
3. Small white onion, 1, diced
4. Tomato paste, 2 T
5. Beef broth, low sodium, 1 c
6. Paprika, .5 tsp.
7. Cumin, 1 tsp.
8. Chili powder, 2 tsp.
9. Olive oil, 2 tsp.
10. Chuck tender roast, 2 lbs.

What You Do:

1. Place paprika, cumin, and chili powder into a small bowl and mix everything together. Rub this mixture into the chuck roast. Make sure that you cover the chuck roast well.
2. Place a large skillet on top of the stove and warm it to medium high. Add in the olive oil and let it get hot. Place beef into the skillet and sear for two minutes. Turn the roast and sear every side. Take the beef out of the skillet and put into the bottom of slow cooker.
3. Add the diced onion into the skillet you seared the beef in and cook for three minutes until onions become soft and translucent. Add garlic and cook until fragrant. Pour the beef broth into the skillet and scrape with a wooden spoon to deglaze the pan.

4. Add the minced chipotle and tomato paste into the skillet and, using a whisk, stir until everything is combined. Bring to boil, lower the heat to a simmer and simmer for five minutes until sauce has thickened. Take off heat and pour over beef in bottom of slow cooker.

5. Place lid on slow cooker and set on low. Cook for eight hours until the beef will shred easily with a fork.

6. When beef is done, take out of slow cooker and shred with two forks. Place back into the slow cooker and stir to coat with juices.

7. Use as you would any meat mixture in your favorite Mexican dishes or eat as is.

Chipotle Steak Salad (Low Carb)

4 – servings

What You Need:

1. Reduced fat cheddar cheese, .5 c, shredded
2. Chopped cilantro, 1 T
3. Sliced avocado, .5
4. Diced and seeded tomato, 1
5. Washed and torn, romaine lettuce, 1 head
6. Taco seasoning packet, .5
7. Lean steaks, 4
8. Toppings of choice

What You Do:

1. Begin by heating a grill or grill pan to medium. Rub the taco seasoning into the meat, making sure it is well coated. Set this aside to let it marinate.
2. Once your grill is hot, place steaks on the grill and cook for 5 minutes per side until done to the desired doneness.
3. Take off the grill and place on cutting board. Allow to rest about 4 minutes.
4. While steaks are cooking, wash and tear lettuce. Divide out among 4 plates.
5. Slice the steaks across the grain and add on top of the lettuce. Add avocado, tomato, and cilantro. Sprinkle with cheese. Use salsa as the salad dressing if you would like to. Enjoy.

Chile Relleno Casserole (Low Carb)

4 – servings

What You Need:

For topping:
1. Salt
2. Mexican blend cheese, shredded, 1 c
3. Diced green chilies, 7 oz.
4. Flour, 2 T
5. Milk, .75 c
6. Eggs, 2

For beef mixture:
1. Taco seasoning, 1 T
2. Ground beef, 1 lb.

What You Do:
1. The first thing you need to do is preheat your oven to 350.
2. Place a skillet on the stove and heat to medium high. Add in the ground beef and allow it to cook until it is completely browned.
3. Make sure you break the beef into smaller pieces as it cooks up. If the beef accumulates any grease as it cooks, make sure to drain it all off. Add taco seasoning and stir well to combine.
4. Use cooking spray and spray an 8 X 8 pan. Place seasoned ground beef in bottom of the pan.
5. Crack the eggs into a bowl and add flour and milk. Whisk until there aren't any lumps left in the mixture. Add in the cheese and green chilies. Stir with a spoon until well combined
6. Pour egg mixture over ground beef mixture and put in the preheated oven. Bake for 20 minutes until top is golden brown.

Steak and Mushroom Fajita Sandwiches

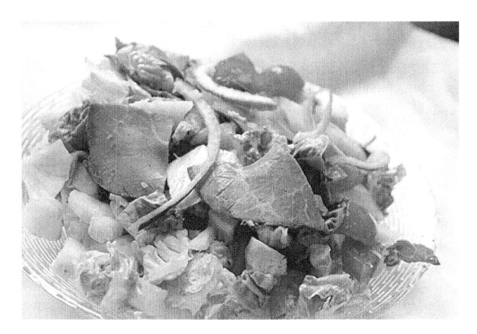

4 – servings

What You Need:

1. Fat free sour cream, .25 c
2. Romaine lettuce leaves, torn, 4
3. Whole wheat tortillas, 4
4. Salt
5. Pepper
6. Dried oregano, 2 tsp.
7. Beef sirloin tip steak, 1 lb., cut into strips
8. Medium red bell pepper, 1, cut into strips
9. Minced garlic, 2 cloves
10. Medium red onion, 1, sliced into strips
11. Olive oil, 1 T plus 2 tsp.

What You Do:

1. The first thing you need to do is warm your oven to 350 degrees.

2. Place a large skillet on top of your stove and warm it to medium high heat. Add one T olive oil and allow to warm up.

3. Put mushroom into the skillet and cook about 6 minutes until softened. Add bell peppers, garlic, and onions. Continue to cook until peppers and onions are softened. This should take about 4 minutes.

4. Add in beef and lower the heat to medium. Cook about 10 minutes until beef is no longer pink. Sprinkle with oregano, pepper, and salt. Stir everything together really well to make sure that all of the seasonings are evenly distributed.

5. Lower the heat to a simmer and cover. Let the mixture simmer about 5 minutes. Drain mixture if you find that it has accumulated any fat.

6. Stack the tortillas together and wrap them in aluminum foil. Place on baking sheet and put in the oven for about 15 minutes to warm. Take tortillas out of the oven and carefully unwrap.

7. Divide the meat mixture among the four tortillas and top with lettuce and sour cream if desired. Enjoy.

Pork and Black Bean Stew (Dairy Free)

4 – servings

What You Need:

1. No salt added black beans, drained and rinsed, 14.5 oz. can
2. No salt added diced tomatoes in juice, 14.5 oz. can
3. No salt added chicken broth, 14 oz. can
4. Taco seasoning packet, 1
5. Cumin, 1 tsp.
6. Minced chipotle pepper in adobo sauce, 2 peppers
7. Adobo sauce, 1 tsp.
8. Garlic, 3 cloves
9. Chopped onions, 1.25 c
10. Pork loin, 1 lb., fat trimmed, cut into one inch cubes
11. Extra virgin olive oil, 2 tsp.
12. Crushed red pepper flakes, 1 tsp., optional

What You Do:

1. Place a Dutch oven on the stove and allow it to heat up to medium high.
2. Add in the cubed pork and allow the meat to cook for about six minutes, stirring occasionally until all sides have been browned.
3. Add in the garlic and onion and cook for three minutes until the onions begin to soften. Add taco seasoning, cumin, adobo sauce, and chipotle peppers and mix well to combine.

4. Place red pepper flakes, if using, beans, tomatoes, and broth into the pot. Stir well to combine. Bring the pot to a boil and then turn the heat down to low.

5. Place lid on pot and simmer between 45 minutes to an hour. Once pork is tender, remove from pot and shred with two forks. Return to pot and stir to combine.

6. Divide stew out into bowls. You can serve this over rice if you would like to.

Poultry

Chicken Skillet

4 – servings

What You Need:

1. Chopped cilantro, 1 T
2. Quartered cherry tomatoes, 1 c
3. Green enchilada cause, 15 oz. can
4. Black beans, rinsed, 1 c
5. Skinless, boneless chicken breasts, 1 lb.
6. Crumbled queso fresco, 4 tsp.

What You Do:

1. Place a skillet on the stove and heat it up to medium high. Spray the heated pan with olive oil cooking spray.
2. Sprinkle both sides of the chicken breasts with pepper and salt. Place into heated skillet and cook until browned on both sides.
3. Place the black beans into the skillet and allow to heat up for about two minutes. Add the green enchilada sauce and stir well. Allow this mixture to come to a boil. Turn the heat down to a simmer.
4. Place a lid on the skillet and simmer until the internal temperature of the chicken has reached 160. This should take about 20 minutes.
5. Add the cilantro and cherry tomatoes and stir well to distribute. Divide evenly onto plates. Top each serving with one tsp. of crumbled queso fresco. Enjoy.

Salsa Verde Stuffed Poblanos (Low Carb, Dairy Free)

4 – servings

What You Need:

1. Frozen riced cauliflower, 10 oz. bag
2. 93% lean ground turkey, 1 lb.
3. Diced white onion, .5 c
4. Lime juice, .5 of a lime
5. Cilantro leaves, 1 c
6. Tomatillos, 11 oz. can
7. Poblano peppers halved and seeded 4

What You Do:

1. The first thing you need to do is heat your oven to 350.
2. Add water to a large pot and bring to a boil. Add the cleaned pepper halves to the pot and let them soften. This will take about eight minutes.
3. Place lime juice, cilantro, and tomatillos into a blender. Blend until completely smooth.
4. Place a large skillet and warm it up over medium high heat. Add the diced onion and cook for about one minute until softened. Add turkey and cook until browned. Breaking it up as it cooks. If the meat needs to be drained, drain it now.
5. While the turkey is cooking, cook the cauliflower in the microwave for three minutes.
6. Add the steamed cauliflower to the turkey and onions in the skillet along with .66 c of the tomatillo mix out of the blender. Stir well to combine and let everything cook an additional minute.

7. Pour .5 c of the tomatillo mix into the bottom of a casserole dish. Place the poblano halves onto the tomatillo mixture. Spoon the meat mixture evenly onto each pepper half until all mixture is used up.
8. Put casserole dish into the preheated oven and bake for 20 minutes.
9. Take out of the oven and allow to cool a bit before serving.
10. Serve and enjoy.

Taco Casserole (Low Carb)

10 – servings

What You Need:

1. 2% shredded cheddar cheese, .66 c
2. Diced tomatoes, drained, 15 oz. can
3. 2% cottage cheese, 1 c
4. Taco seasoning, 1 packet
5. 93% lean ground turkey, 2 lbs.

What You Do:

1. The first thing you need to do is warm your oven to 400.
2. Place a skillet on the stove and heat to medium high. Add in the ground turkey and allow it to cook until it is completely browned.
3. Make sure that you break the turkey apart as it cooks. If there is any grease that accumulates, make sure that you drain it off.
4. Add a half of a c of water to turkey and add in the taco seasoning packet. Let simmer for about ten minutes until water has been absorbed. Once the mixture is done, place in the bottom of an 8 X 8 casserole dish.
5. Place the tomatoes, cottage cheese, and shredded cheese into a bowl and mix well. Pour on top of the meat mixture. Place in oven and bake for about 20 minutes until golden brown and bubbly.
6. Serve and enjoy.

Chili Lime Jalapeno Turkey Burgers (Low Carb, Dairy Free)

8 – servings

What You Need:

1. Egg white, 1
2. Sea salt
3. Lime juice, 2 T
4. Diced green onions, 2 T
5. Seeded and chopped jalapeno, 1 small
6. 93 % lean ground turkey, 1 lb.
7. Toppings of choice:
8. Spinach
9. Tomato slices

What You Do:

1. Place a nonstick grill pan on the stove and heat to medium high.
2. While the grill pan is heating, chop the green onions and jalapeno very finely.
3. Place the egg white, salt, lime juice, green onion, garlic, jalapeno, and turkey into a bowl.
4. Using your hands, mix well until everything is combined. Divide out into eight portions and form into eight patties.
5. Cook the burgers in batches. Place the burgers onto the preheated grill pan. Cook the burgers for one minute to sear one side.
6. Cover with a large lid in order to keep the steam in and keep the burger moist. Only do this after the first side has been

seared. Cook under the lid for four minutes. Turn burger over and repeat on the other side.

7. Check the internal temperature of the burger. Make sure the internal temperature has reached 165.
8. Once cooked thoroughly, place on plates and add your toppings of choice. Serve and enjoy.

Cilantro Lime Chicken with Tomato Relish (Low Carb, Dairy Free)

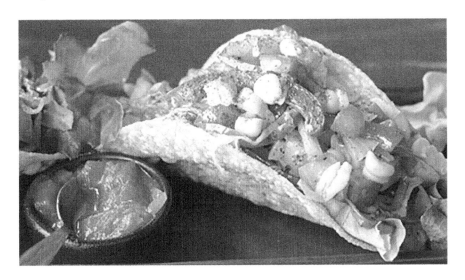

4 – servings

What You Need:

1. Pepper
2. Salt
3. Cumin, 2 tsp.
4. Skinless, boneless chicken breast tenders, 1 lb.
5. Halved cherry tomatoes, 10
6. Lime juice, .5 of a lime
7. Chopped cilantro, 2 T
8. Chopped green onions, 3

What You Do:

1. Put the tomatoes, lime juice, cilantro, and green onions into a medium bowl. Cover the bowl and place it into the refrigerator until ready to use. The lets the flavors marinate and get happy.

2. Place the chicken on a plate and season all sides with pepper, salt, and cumin.
3. Place a skillet on the stove and heat to medium high. You might have to cook these in batches. Place some chicken into the heated skillet and cook five minutes on each side. Make sure that you check the chicken's internal temperature and make sure that it comes up to 165. Remove from skillet and place on a plate. Make sure to keep it warm.
4. Continue cooking chicken until all tenders have been cooked to an internal temperature of 165.
5. When all the chicken tenders are done, place on a plate and top with the tomato-lime relish. Serve and enjoy.

Turkey Skillet with Salsa and Eggs (Low Carb, Dairy Free)

4 – servings

What You Need:

1. Pepper
2. Salt
3. Cumin, .5 tsp.
4. Large eggs, 4
5. Salsa, 16 oz. jar
6. 93% lean ground turkey, 1 lb.

What You Do:

1. Place a skillet on the stove and heat to medium high. Add in the ground turkey and allow it to cook until it is completely browned.
2. As the turkey is cooking, make sure that you break it into smaller pieces. If accumulates any fat, make sure that you drain it off before continuing.
3. Add the salsa to the skillet along with the cumin and stir well to combine everything. Bring to a boil. Turn heat down to low and simmer. Make four well in the mixture to hold each egg.
4. Crack one egg into each well. Sprinkle tops of eggs with pepper and salt. Cover skillet with a lid. Continue to simmer for about eight minutes until eggs have set up to the desired doneness.
5. Take off heat and cool for a bit. Serve and enjoy.

Chicken Chili with Jalapeno and Cheddar (Low Carb)

4 – servings

What You Need:

1. Diced carrots, 1 c
2. Shredded pepper jack cheese, .5 c
3. Low fat cream cheese, .25 c
4. Chicken broth, .5 c
5. Oregano, 1 tsp.
6. Chili powder, 1 T
7. Cumin, 1 T
8. Diced jarred jalapeno slices, .33 c
9. Skinless, boneless chicken breast, 1 lb.

What You Do:

1. Spray a Dutch oven with cooking spray. Place the Dutch oven on the stove and heat to medium high.
2. Add in the diced chicken along with the diced jalapenos. Cook until chicken turns opaque.
3. Add oregano, chili powder, and cumin to the chicken and jalapenos. Stir to combine and cook for one minute.
4. Add carrots and chicken broth. Stir to combine. Bring to a boil. Once boiling, turn heat down to low and cover.
5. Allow this mixture to simmer for 20 minutes until the carrots are soft.
6. Add in pepper jack and cream cheese. Stir until mixed well and cheese is melted. Allow to simmer for five minutes more.
7. Divide evenly into bowls.
8. Serve and enjoy.

Soft Mexican Chicken Salad (Low Carb, Dairy Free)

2 – servings

What You Need:

1. Juice from jarred salsa, 2 tsp.
2. Taco seasoning, 1 tsp.
3. Light mayonnaise, 1 T
4. Canned chicken, drained, 1 c

What You Do:

1. Put the drained chicken in a bowl. Take a fork and break the chicken into small pieces.
2. Add the mayonnaise to the chicken and combine well. Mash the chicken into the mayonnaise with the fork.
3. Add the salsa juice and taco seasoning into chicken mixture and continue to mash until everything is well combined. Serve and enjoy.

Grilled Chicken with Pico de Gallo (Low Carb, Dairy Free)

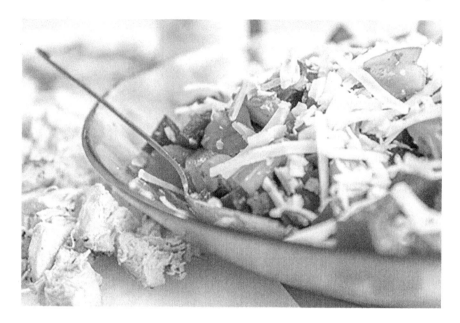

4 – servings

What You Need:

1. Minced garlic, 1 clove
2. Diced jalapeno pepper, 1
3. Diced onion, .5 c
4. Seeded and diced Roma tomatoes, 4
5. Pepper
6. Salt
7. Limes, 2
8. Cilantro, 1 bunch
9. Skinless, boneless chicken breast tenders, 1 lb.

What You Do:

1. Place a nonstick grill pan on top of stove and heat to medium high or preheat a regular grill.
2. Place one tsp. salt, juice of one lime, and one c chopped cilantro in a shallow dish. Stir to combine. Add the chicken and stir to coat. Set aside and let marinade for at least 15 minutes.
3. While the chicken is marinating, dice up the garlic, onions, a handful of cilantro, jalapeno, and tomatoes. Mix well to combine all flavors.
4. Add in some pepper and salt. Add in the juice of the other lime and mix again to combine everything. Set aside until ready to serve.
5. Take the chicken out of the marinade and place on the preheated grill or grill pan.
6. Cook chicken for five minutes on each side until internal temperature reaches 165. When cooked through, place chicken tenders on plate and top with the Pico de Gallo mixture.

Turkey Taco Meatballs (Low Carb)

6 – servings

What You Need:

1. Chopped cilantro
2. 2% cheddar cheese, 12 cubes
3. Taco seasoning, 1 packet
4. Chopped garlic, 1 T
5. Eggs, 2
6. Chopped green onions, .5 c
7. 93% lean ground turkey, 1 lb.

What You Do:

1. The first thing you need to do is warm your oven to 425.
2. Crack the eggs into a bowl and beat them slightly. Add garlic, green onions, taco seasonings, and turkey.
3. Using your hands, mix until everything is combined well. Divide the turkey mixture into six even balls.
4. Take one cheese cube and press into the center of a turkey ball. Make sure the cheese is completely encased with the turkey.
5. Line a baking sheet with foil and spray with cooking spray. Put into preheated oven and bake for ten minutes until golden brown.
6. Sprinkle with chopped cilantro and shredded cheese.
7. Serve and enjoy.

Slow cooker Salsa Chicken (Low Carb)

6 – servings

What You Need:

1. Reduced fat sour cream, .5 c
2. Can of reduced fat cream of mushroom soup
3. Packed of reduced sodium taco seasoning
4. Salsa, 1 c
5. Skinless and boneless chicken breasts, 4

What You Do:

1. Place all of the chicken to the bottom of your slow cooker. Top the chicken with the taco seasoning pack.
2. If you want, you can rub the seasoning into the chicken and allow it to marinade for a bit before placing it in your slow cooker.
3. Pour the mushroom soup and salsa over the chicken. Place the lid on your slow cooker and set the machine to cook for six to eight hours on low.
4. Remove the chicken from the slow cooker and shred it. Place it back in, making sure the heat is off to the pot, and mix in the shredded chicken along with the sour cream.
5. If you want to reduce the sodium content in the recipe, even more, you can just use half of the taco seasoning packet.

Slow Cooker Chicken Fajitas

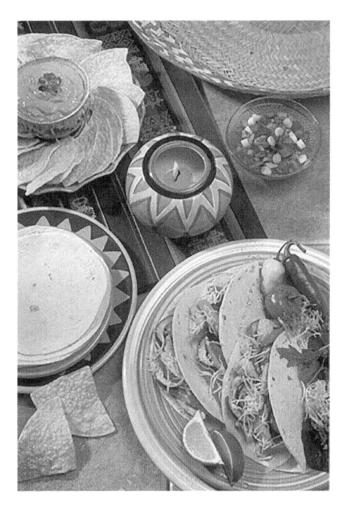

4 – servings

What You Need:

1. Fajita toppings – salsa, guacamole, low-fat shredded cheese, light sour cream
2. Package low fat or low carb fajita tortillas
3. Package fajita seasoning
4. Bell peppers, 2

5. Yellow onion
6. Skinless and boneless chicken breasts, 1 lb.

What You Do:

1. Cut open the peppers and remove the ribs and seeds. Slice up the peppers and onion into a quarter inch thickness.
2. Separate out the onion layers into individual slices. Lay out the peppers and onions in the bottom of your slow cooker.
3. Add the chicken breasts on top of the peppers and onions. A good option for the chicken is to use a bag of thin frozen chicken breasts, and don't thaw them beforehand.
4. Season the chicken with the fajita seasoning packet.
5. Sit the lid on the slow cooker and allow the chicken to cook on high for three to four hours. You can also cook it on low for six to eight hours.
6. Once the chicken has cooked all the way through, and the vegetables have become tender, take the chicken out of the slow cooker. You can either cut them into strips or shred them up.
7. Now you can assemble your fajitas. Warm the tortillas before assembling so that they are easier to fold.
8. Top the chicken with you favorite toppings. For more filling protein, you can add some fat-free refried beans.
9. You can add any leftover chicken back into the juices and then store in an air tight container in the fridge. This will keep the chicken moist, and it reheats nicely.

Slow cooker Tex Mex Chicken (Dairy Free)

6 – servings

What You Need:

1. Chopped cilantro for topping
2. Rinsed black beans, 15 oz.
3. Salsa, 10 oz.
4. Packet taco seasoning
5. Skinless and boneless chicken breasts, 1 lb.

What You Do:

1. To make clean up a lot easier, place a slow cooker liner bag into your slow cooker.
2. Place all of the chicken ingredients, except for the cilantro, into your slow cooker. Mix everything together to make sure that the chicken is well coated.
3. Place the lid on your slow cooker all it to cook for six and a half hours on low.
4. Once the chicken is cooked all the way through, remove the chicken from the pot and shred it up with two forks.
5. Stir the shredded chicken back into the mixture. Use a slotted spoon and remove the chicken and place it in a blow.
6. Top the cooked chicken with cilantro if you would like and enjoy.

Spinach and Chicken Flautas

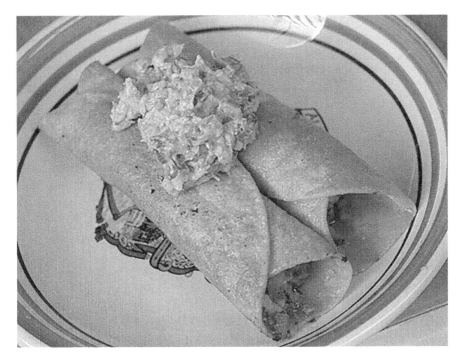

10 – servings

What You Need:

1. Salsa – serving
2. Olive oil, 1 tsp.
3. Shredded soft cheese like Monterey jack, 6 oz.
4. Burrito sized flour tortillas, 5
5. Chopped baby spinach, 3 c
6. Minced jalapeno pepper
7. Chili powder, 1 tsp.
8. Ground cumin, 1 tsp.
9. Garlic powder, 1 tsp.
10. Salt, 1 tsp.

11. Paprika, 1 tsp.
12. Water, 2 c
13. Chicken broth, 16 oz.
14. Skinless and boneless chicken thighs, 1 lb.

What You Do:

1. Start out by heating up your oven to 450.
2. Place the chicken thighs into a sauté pan that has deep sides and cover the chicken with the water.
3. Place the pan on medium high and allow the water to come up to a boil. Turn the heat down so that the water simmers for 20 minutes.
4. Take the chicken out of the water and shred it up.
5. Mix together the paprika, salt, garlic powder, ground cumin, and chili powder in a large bowl and in the toss in the shredded chicken.
6. Reserve a quarter c of the water that you cooked the chicken in. Add this to a pot and mix in the spinach and jalapeno and allow them to cook over low until the spinach has wilted. This should take about two to three minutes.
7. Slice your tortillas in half.
8. Place a tenth of the chicken mixture, around a T, along with the long edge of your tortilla.
9. Add a tenth of the spinach mixture and then the cheese on top of the chicken.
10. Roll up the tortilla, starting along the straight edge.
11. Lay the rolled up chicken seam-side down onto an oiled baking sheet. Continue this with the rest of the tortillas and filling mixtures.

12. Brush the tops of your flautas with some olive oil, or you can spritz them with some cooking spray.
13. Place them in the oven and let them bake for ten minutes.
14. Flip over the flautas and then cook them for another ten minutes, or until they crisp up. Serve them with your favorite salsa or guacamole.

Slow cooker Chicken Enchiladas

6 – servings

What You Need:

1. Medium whole grain tortillas, 6 (make sure they are not corn because they tend to fall apart easily)
2. Fat free sour cream, 8 oz.
3. Reduced fat shredded cheddar cheese, 1.5 c
4. Pepper, .5 tsp.
5. Chili powder, 1 tsp.
6. Cumin, 1 tsp.
7. Garlic powder, .5 tsp.
8. Can of jalapenos, 4 oz.
9. No sugar added red enchilada sauce, 16 oz.
10. Skinless chicken breast filets, 2

What You Do:

1. Start by setting the oven to 350.
2. Cover a baking dish with aluminum foil and lay the chicken in the bottom of the dish.
3. Place the chicken in the oven and cook until the juices start to run clear when you piece it with a fork. This should take about 35 to 45 minutes.
4. If you chicken had skin on it, remove the skin at this point.
5. Shred up the chicken, or you can cut them into bite sized pieces.

6. Grab a decent sized bowl and add in the pepper, chili powder, cumin, garlic powder, and chicken. Add in a pinch of salt, or however much your taste buds say you need.

7. Toss everything together until the chicken is well coated in the seasonings.

8. To this mixture, add a c of cheese, a half c of sour cream, a half c of enchilada sauce, and jalapeno pepper. Mix everything together so that everything is well distributed.

9. Add a half c of the chicken mixture onto the center of every tortilla. Make sure that you leave around two inches at the bottom of the tortilla clean and fold the tortilla over the filling.

10. Continue folding until you have finished all of the enchiladas.

11. Stack all of your enchiladas into your slow cooker. Add some of the enchilada sauce on top of each of the layers of enchiladas as you stack them in.

12. There will typically be two layers of three enchiladas or three layers of two enchiladas, depending on the size and shape of your slow cooker.

13. Mix the rest of the enchilada sauce with a half a c of sour cream. Pour this mixture over top of the enchilada.

14. Place the lid on the cooker and allow them to cook for three to four hours on low, or until everything is hot and bubbly.

15. Cut between the enchiladas and carefully take them out, one enchilada at a time, using a large spatula.

16. Using a spoon, pour the liquid that is left in the slow cooker over your enchiladas and sprinkle them with the rest of the cheese.

17. Garnish your enchiladas with shredded lettuce and diced tomatoes.

Creamy Green Chile Enchilada Soup

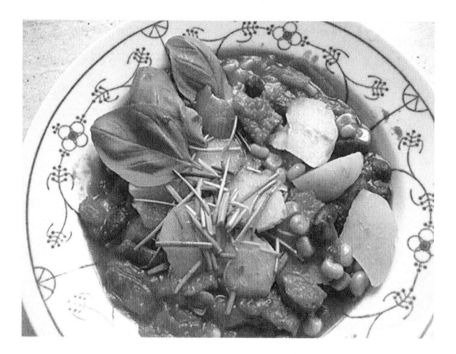

10 – servings

What You Need:

1. Corn starch, 1 T (if needed)
2. Pepper
3. Salt
4. Uncooked instant rice, .75 c
5. Cream cheese, 8 oz.
6. Frozen corn, 1 c
7. Garlic powder, 1 tsp.
8. Onion powder, 1 tsp.
9. Chili powder, 1 T
10. Ground cumin, 2 T

11. Water, .75 c
12. Diced green chilies, 4 oz.
13. Green chili enchilada sauce, 2 cans
14. Chicken breasts, 24 oz.
15. Chicken broth, 32 oz.
16. Optional toppings: sour cream, avocado, and shredded cheese

What You Do:

1. In your slow cooker combine together the cumin, onion powder, garlic powder, chili powder, water, green chilies, green enchilada sauce, and broth.
2. You can adjust any the amounts of seasonings to your taste.
3. Snuggle the chicken breasts into the mixture in the slow cooker and cover the cooker with the lid. Set the cooker to cook for seven hours on low.
4. Once you hit the seven hour mark, take the chicken out of the cooker and place it in another dish.
5. Shred up the chicken and then mix it back into the mixture in the cooker.
6. Mix in the cream cheese, corn, and instant rice to your soup mixture and add the lid back onto the cooker.
7. Place the lid back on and allow the mixture to cook for another 30 minutes.
8. Stir the soup again; making sure that all of the cream cheese is well distributed and melted. You may have to cook the mixture a bit longer to make sure that the cream cheese does get completely melted.
9. Now you need to judge the consistency of the soup in your cooker.

10. If you want the soup to be a bit thicker, you can mix in a T of cornstarch into an eighth of a c of water and then stir this back into your soup. Keep the lid off and allow the soup to thicken for about ten to 20 minutes.

11. If you see that the soup is already thick enough for your taste, you can skip this step.

12. Feel free to use chicken thighs in this recipe if you want a little extra flavor. The important thing to remember to do is to make sure you remove as much fat from the thighs as you can before you start to cook anything.

Chicken Avocado Casserole (Low Carb)

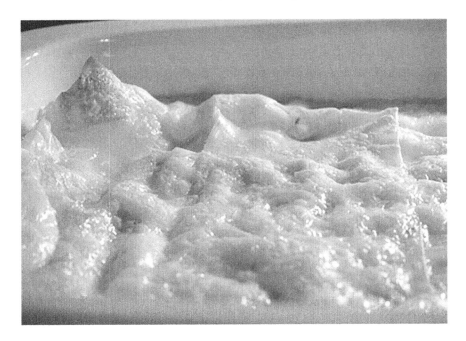

6 – servings

What You Need:

1. Pepper
2. Salt
3. Frank's red hot, 1 T
4. Shredded cheddar cheese, 8 oz.
5. Sour cream, 8 oz.
6. Medium pepper
7. Medium onion
8. Avocados, 4
9. Cooked boneless chicken thighs, 8

What You Do:

1. Start out by setting your oven to 350.
2. Begin by cooking your chicken thighs. You can do this by baking you chicken at 350 for about an hour and a half, or until the internal temperature reaches 165.
3. You can also cube up the chicken and pan fry it until the juices run clear. Once the chicken is cooked through, allow it to cool off completely and then shred it into smaller pieces if needed.
4. Carefully slice the avocados in half and remove the pit. Try to scoop the avocado halves out whole and then slice them into thin strips.
5. You can also slice them into strips while they are still in the skin and the scoop out the slices
6. Grease up a baking dish with some nonstick spray and line the avocado slices into the bottom of the dish.
7. If you have any avocado slices leftover, reserve them for later use.
8. To keep them from oxidizing and turning brown, coat them with some lemon or lime juice.
9. Slice up the onions and peppers and place them in a hot pan and fry them up until the onions have caramelized.
10. Place the chicken into a bowl and add in any of the remaining avocado that didn't fit in the bottom of the baking dish as well as the pepper, onion, sour cream, cheddar cheese, hot sauce, pepper, and salt. Adjust any of the flavorings as you need.
11. Spoon the chicken mixture into the baking dish on top of the avocado slices. Place this in your oven and let it cook for 20 minutes. Slice into six squares and enjoy.

Seafood

Spicy Shrimp Burrito Bowl (Dairy Free)

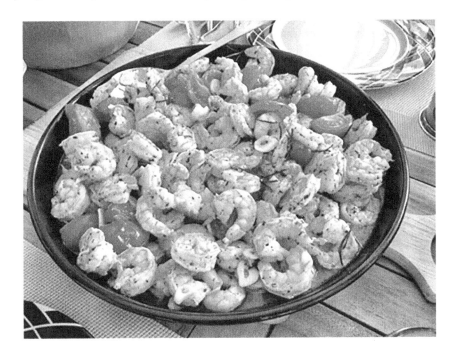

4 – servings

What You Need:

Salsa:

1. Jalapeno pepper
2. Salt, 1 tsp.
3. Fresh cilantro, 1 c

4. Juice of a lime
5. Minced garlic, 2 cloves
6. Roma tomatoes, 6
7. Cilantro Lime Rice:
8. Sea salt, .25 tsp.
9. Fresh lime juice, 1 T
10. Chopped cilantro, 1.5 T
11. Bag frozen riced cauliflower, 10 oz.

Spicy Shrimp:

1. Easy to peel shrimp, 1 lb.
2. Garlic powder, .25 tsp.
3. Cumin, 2 tsp.
4. Mexican chili powder, 2 tsp.

What You Do:

1. Spicy Shrimp:
2. Mix all of the shrimp seasonings together.
3. Place the cleaned shrimp in and toss them together until they are well coated.
4. Place a large pan onto medium high and allow it to heat up.
5. Place the shrimp in your preheated pan. Make sure you work in batches so that your pan never gets too overcrowded.
6. Allow the shrimp to cook until it turns opaque and pink.
7. The raw shrimp will appear translucent and grey. As the shrimp are cooking make sure that you stir it frequently until the

shrimp no longer appears grey and it is completely opaque and pink.

8. This should take around five minutes depending on your shrimp's size and how many you place in your pan at a time.
9. Take the shrimp out and cover them to keep them warm while you are assembling your bowl.
10. Cilantro Lime Rice:
11. Follow the steaming directions on your pack of cauliflower rice.
12. As the cauliflower is cooking, chop up the cilantro.
13. Take the cauliflower out of the microwave and open the bag to release all of the steam.
14. Pour the cooked cauliflower into a bowl and mix in the salt, lime juice, and cilantro. Allow all of the flavors to combine.
15. Salsa:
16. Cut all of your Roma tomatoes in half.
17. Slice up and deseed the jalapeno.
18. Place all of the salsa ingredients into your food processor. If you don't have a food processor you can also us a blender to mix up the salsa.
19. Pulse the mixture until it is finely diced and well combined. This is also a perfect topping for veggies or any other lean protein source.
20. Divide your cauliflower rice between four bowls and top each of the bowls with the cooked shrimp. Top each of the bowls with a quarter c of the salsa mixture.
21. Enjoy.

Shrimp Tacos (Dairy Free)

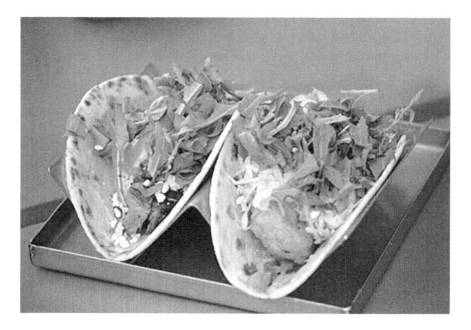

6 – servings

What You Need:

1. Corn tortillas, 6
2. Salt, .25 tsp.
3. Deveined and peeled shrimp, 1 lb.
4. Red pepper flakes, .25 tsp.
5. Paprika, .25 tsp.
6. Ground cumin, .25 tsp.
7. Juice of a lime
8. Olive oil, 1 T

What You Do:

1. Mix together the red pepper, paprika, cumin, lime juice, and olive oil until they are well combined.
2. Add the shrimp to a Ziploc bag and pour in the marinade mixture. Seal up the bag and shake everything together to coat the shrimp.
3. Allow this to sit for 15 minutes to marinade the shrimp.
4. Take the shrimp from the bag and discard any of the remaining marinade.
5. Place a grill pan on medium high and allow it to heat up.
6. Top the shrimp with a sprinkle of salt and then arrange half of them in the heated pan.
7. Allow them to grill for two minutes before flipping, and then grill for another two minutes, or until pink.
8. Take the shrimp off the grill and keep warm.
9. Repeat this with the remaining shrimp.
10. Warm your tortillas and divide the shrimp between them.
11. You can top the shrimp with some homemade salsa if you would like.

Chipotle and Garlic Shrimp (Dairy Free, Low Carb)

1 – servings

What You Need:

1. Garlic seasoning, 2 T
2. Small shrimp, 1 c
3. Chipotle sauce, 3 T

What You Do:

1. Toss your shrimp with some oil until they are well coated and then sprinkle on the garlic seasoning.
2. Make sure that the shrimp are evenly coated with the garlic.
3. Place this in a griddle pan and allow them to cook for around three minutes on both sides, or until the shrimp has turned pink and opaque.
4. Take the shrimp off the once they are cooked through and drizzle them with the chipotle sauce. Sprinkle a little extra garlic over them if you would like.

Salmon with Mexican Rice Salad (Dairy Free)

4 – servings

What You Need:

1. A handful of basil, chopped
2. Wild Alaskan salmon fillets, 4 .25 lb. fillets
3. Handful chopped parsley
4. Low-fat nonstick spray
5. Pepper
6. Salt
7. Small eggplant, cubed
8. Cubed red pepper, .5 pepper
9. Cubed zucchini, .5 zucchini
10. Dry green lentils, .25 c
11. Dry long grain rice, .75 c
12. Dressing:
13. Pinch pepper
14. Salt, .5 tsp.
15. Juice of two limes
16. Extra virgin olive oil, .33 c

What You Do:

1. Dressing:
2. Add all of the dressing ingredients to a bowl and whisk together until they are well combined. If you can handle some heat, you can also whisk in a few shakes of Tabasco sauce.

3. Salmon and Rice:
4. Start out by placing your oven at 400.
5. Add two and a half c of water to a pot and salt it slightly.
6. Allow the water to come to a boil and add in the lentils and rice.
7. Place a lid on the pot and allow the water to come back up to a boil.
8. Turn the heat down and allow them to cook for 20 to 25 minutes until the rice is completely cooked.
9. Drain off the remaining water and allow the lentils and rice to cool.
10. As the rice is cooking, spread the cubed eggplant, red pepper, and zucchini out on a baking sheet. Season them with your favorite flavors.
11. To keep with the Mexican theme, you could use some low-sodium taco seasoning. Spray them with a liberal amount of nonstick spray.
12. Place them in the oven and allow them to cook for 25 to 30 minutes, or until they are tender.
13. Place the cooled rice mixture, the dressing you made earlier, parsley, and roasted vegetables in a bowl and toss them together.
14. Get the salmon ready by spraying it with some low-fat cooking spray and then sprinkle it with basil.
15. Cook the salmon, skin-side down, over medium high, flipping after three minutes.
16. The salmon will easily flake when it is cooked through.
17. Serve the salmon along with the rice salad.

Pacific Cod with Fajita Vegetables (Dairy Free)

4 – servings

What You Need:

1. Pepper
2. Salt
3. Large julienned carrot
4. Sliced yellow bell pepper, 2
5. Sliced red bell pepper, 2
6. Low-fat nonstick spray
7. Scallions, 6
8. Juice and zest of a lime
9. Wild Alaskan Pacific cod, 4 6 oz. fillets

What You Do:

1. Start out by heating up your grill or broiler.
2. Place some aluminum foil over the grill rack and place the cod fillets on top.
3. Top the fillets with the lime juice, zest, and some slices of the scallions.
4. Allow them to grill or broil for six to eight minutes, or until it is cooked all the way through. The fish will turn opaque and will easily flake once it is cooked through.
5. As the fish cooks, spray a large skillet with some low-fat nonstick spray and allow it to heat up for a few moments on high.
6. Add in the bell peppers, the rest of the scallions, and carrot.

7. Allow them to cook, stirring often, for three to five minutes.
8. Divide your cooked veggies between four different plates and top each of them with a cod fillet.
9. Season the top of the fish with some pepper and salt to taste.

Lemon Garlic Shrimp (Dairy Free)

4 – servings

What You Need:

1. Cooked Mexican rice for serving
2. Minced garlic, 5 cloves
3. Cleaned and deveined medium shrimp, 1 lb.
4. Butter, 2 T
5. Pepper
6. Salt
7. Thyme sprigs, 3 to 4
8. Zest of a lemon
9. Thin lemon slices, .5 lemon
10. Lemon wedges, .5 lemon
11. Olive oil, .33 c

What You Do:

1. Start out by heating your oven 400.
2. Grab an eight by eight glass baking dish and mix together the thyme, lemon zest, and olive oil. Make sure that you only add the thyme leaves, not the whole sprig.
3. Make sure that the olive oil covers the bottom of the baking dish. If it doesn't, make sure that you drizzle in some more until the bottom is well covered.
4. Sprinkle in some pepper and salt to the oil mixture. Bake this mixture in the oven for 10 to 12 minutes.

5. Make sure you check it every few minutes to ensure that the oil isn't getting too brown. If it starts to brown up too quickly, take it out.
6. Mix in the butter, stirring to allow it to melt completely.
7. Add in the thinly sliced lemons, don't squeeze, garlic, and shrimp.
8. Toss everything so that it is all coated in the oil mixture.
9. Allow this mixture to bake for eight to ten minutes or until the shrimp has turned pink and it had just started to curl up, so make sure you check on it often.
10. Serve the cooked shrimp over top of some Mexican rice.
11. Toss it with a little extra EVOO and serve with the lemon wedges.

Tilapia Veracruz (Dairy Free, Low Carb)

6 – servings

What You Need:

1. Lime
2. Capers, 2 T
3. Green olives, .25 c
4. Tomatoes, 2 c
5. Chopped oregano, .5 tsp.
6. Bay leaves, 2
7. Sliced garlic, 3 cloves
8. Sliced Anaheim chili
9. Sliced onion
10. Salt
11. Tilapia fillets, 6
12. Extra virgin olive oil, 2 T

What You Do:

1. Place the oil in a large pan and allow it to heat on medium high.
2. Season both sides of the all the fish fillets with some pepper and salt. Make sure you lightly press the seasonings in with your fingers.
3. Place the fish into your hot skillet and allow them to cook until they are golden brown on the bottom. This should take three to four minutes.
4. Flip the fish carefully and allow it to cook for another two minutes.

5. Take the fish out and set it on a plate while you cook everything else.

6. Add the chili and the onion to your skillet and sauté it for two to three minutes or until the onions have softened.

7. Mix in the garlic and cook it for 30 seconds.

8. Mix in the capers, green olives, crushed tomatoes, oregano, and bay leaves into the mixtures. Allow this to come to a simmer and cook until it has thickened slightly, around five minutes.

9. Place the fish back into your pan and let it simmer for three to four minutes more, or until the fish has cooked all the way through.

10. The fish should be opaque and should easily flake once cooked through. Take the bay leaves out of the mixture. Serve with a lime wedge.

11. Oven Method:

12. Place your oven at 350.

13. Add the oil to the bottom of a 9 by 13 baking dish.

14. Place the fillets in the bottom of the pan. Frozen fillets work best for this cooking method.

15. Place all the remaining ingredients on top of the fish, minus the lime wedge.

16. Allow this mixture to cook until the fish flakes easily with a fork. This should take between 20 to 30 minutes.

Salmon with Summer Salsa (Dairy Free)

4 – servings

What You Need:
1. Lime wedges
2. Chopped cilantro, .25 c
3. Pepper
4. Salt
5. Minced red onion, .25 c
6. Cooked corn kernels, .5 c
7. Olive oil, 1 tsp.
8. Balsamic vinegar, 1 T
9. Crushed garlic clove
10. Chopped avocado, .5 avocado
11. Chopped tomato, 1 c
12. Skinless salmon, 4, 4 oz. fillets

What You Do:
1. Start by setting your oven to 325 degrees.
2. Mix all of the ingredients together, except for the lime and salmon.
3. Allow the mixture to refrigerate for around 30 minutes so that all of the flavors can meld together.
4. Place the salmon in your preheated oven and allow it to cook for 15 to 20 minutes, or until it has cooked all the way through. The salmon should flake easily and should be opaque when it is fully cooked.
5. Serve the cooked salmon topped with the salsa and lime wedge. A great summer option is to allow the salmon to cool off completely after it has cooked. Serving cool salmon with the chilled salsa is delicious.

Vegetables

Cilantro Lime Cauliflower Rice (Dairy Free, Low Carb)

4 – servings

What You Need:

1. Sea salt, .25 tsp.
2. Fresh lime juice, 1 T
3. Chopped cilantro, 1.5 T
4. Frozen riced cauliflower, 10 oz.

What You Do:

1. Follow the directions on the package of riced cauliflower to cook it.
2. As the cauliflower is cooking, chop up your cilantro.
3. Take the cauliflower out of the microwave and open the bag to allow all of the steam to release. Make sure that you don't get burned.
4. Pour the cooked cauliflower into a bowl and add in the salt, cilantro, and lime juice. Stir everything together to combine all of the flavors.

Sweet Pepper Poppers (Low Carb)

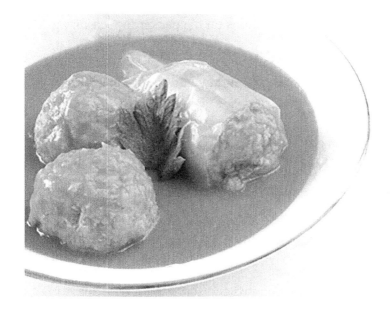

6 – servings

What You Need:

1. Salsa, for serving
2. 2% shredded cheese, .5 c
3. Chopped cilantro, 2 T
4. Taco seasoning packet
5. 93% lean ground turkey, 1 lb.
6. A bag of mini sweet bell peppers

What You Do:

1. Start by halving the peppers and removing their seeds.
2. Set your oven to 350 degrees.
3. While the oven is heating up, brown the ground turkey.

4. Once the turkey is thoroughly cooked, drain off any fat that may have accumulated, and then sprinkle in the taco seasoning packet. Follow the directions on the packet for seasoning.

5. Place the halved bell peppers onto a baking sheet.

6. Ease the ground, seasoned turkey into the bell peppers.

7. Make sure you try to get an even amount of turkey into each bell pepper half.

8. Sprinkle the tops of each of the peppers with some cheese.

9. Place the baking tray in the oven and allow it to cook for five minutes.

10. Allow the peppers to cool slightly and then place over onto a serving plate.

11. Sprinkle them with cilantro and serve them with some salsa for dipping.

Roasted Corn Guacamole

4-6 – servings

What You Need:

1. Pepper
2. Salt
3. Chili pepper, 1 tsp.
4. Garlic powder, 1.5 tsp.
5. Chopped cilantro, .25 c
6. Diced onion, .25 c
7. Diced small tomato
8. Lime juice, 2 tsp.
9. Large avocados, 2-3
10. Cumin, 2 tsp., divided
11. Butter, 1 T
12. An ear of corn

What You Do:

1. Heat up a grill and brush the corn with some butter and sprinkle it with a tsp. of the cumin.
2. Place the corn on the grill and allow it to cook for five minutes. Make sure you turn it often during the cooking process to make sure it browns evenly.
3. The corn should char slightly during the cooking process.
4. Take it off the grill and use a sharp know to cut the kernels off the cob. Set the kernels aside and discard the cob.

5. Pit the avocados and scoop out the meat of the avocados and place it in a bowl.
6. Mash up the avocados using a fork until they are creamy but they still have a little bit of texture.
7. Add in the chili powder, garlic powder, cilantro, and lime juice. Mix all of the ingredients together to make sure everything is evenly distributed.
8. Add in some pepper and salt to taste. Carefully stir in the corn, tomatoes, and onion.
9. Serve the guacamole immediately.
10. This is a great topper for any of the recipes in the beef and poultry sections of this book.

Bean and Spinach Burrito

6 – servings

What You Need:

1. Whole grain tortillas, 6
2. Salt, to taste
3. Fat-free Greek yogurt, 6 T
4. Salsa, .5 c
5. Reduced-fat grated cheddar cheese, .5 c
6. Chopped romaine lettuce, .5 c
7. Cooked Mexican rice, 1.5 c
8. Drained and rinsed black beans, 15 oz.
9. Baby spinach, 6 c

What You Do:

1. Set your oven to 300 degrees.
2. Stack all of the tortillas on top of each other and wrap them in a large piece aluminum foil.
3. Sit the stack of tortillas on a cookie sheet and place them in the heated oven to warm for 15 minutes.
4. Allow them to warm as you prepare the rest of the ingredients.
5. Add the spinach to the food processor and pulse them a few times until they are finely chopped. You can also use a knife to slice up the leaves if you don't have a food processor.
6. Place a large pan on medium and allow it to heat up.
7. Add in the spinach and black beans. Cook the mixture until the spinach has wilted. This should take around three minutes.

8. Evenly distribute this mixture between you six tortillas. Make sure that you leave about two inches on the end of the wrap to aid in folding it up.

9. Add about a quarter c of the mixture to each tortilla and top with the lettuce, salsa, cheese, and the yogurt. Make sure you distribute the toppings evenly among them. Fold the tortilla over and under on the ends.

Stuffed Southwest Style Sweet Potatoes (Dairy Free)

4 – servings

What You Need:

1. Pepper
2. Salt
3. Chopped cilantro, 2 T
4. Frozen corn kernels, .5 c
5. Cooked black beans, .5 c
6. Chopped tomatoes with juices, 1 c
7. Chili powder, .5 tsp.
8. Ground cumin, 1 tsp.
9. Minced garlic, 1 clove
10. Diced red onion, 1 small
11. Olive oil, 1 tsp.
12. Small sweet potatoes, 4

What You Do:

1. Start out by placing your oven to 400 degrees.
2. Sit the sweet potatoes on a cookie sheet and allow them to bake in your heated oven for 30 minutes.
3. Take the potatoes out of the oven and prick them a few times and then place them back in the oven for another 30 minutes, or until they are completely tender and cooked through.
4. As the sweet potatoes are baking, place a pan on medium and allow it to heat up.

5. Add in the olive oil and the onions and allow them to cook for two minutes. The onions should be soft but they should not be translucent.
6. Add in the garlic and allow it to cook for 30 seconds or until you can start to smell the garlic.
7. Mix in the salt, chili powder, and cumin. Mix everything together until well combined. Mix in the cilantro and season the mixture with a bit more pepper and salt.
8. Taste and adjust the flavorings as you need.
9. To serve the potatoes:
10. Take the sweet potatoes out of the oven and slice them down the middle.
11. Fluff the meat inside of the potato up a little and season it with a bit of salt.
12. Divide the filling you just made between the different potatoes.
13. Enjoy.

Vegetable Chili (Dairy Free)

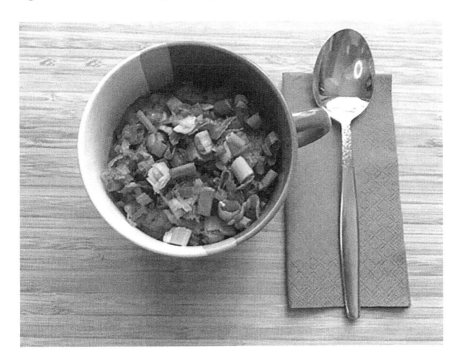

12 – servings

What You Need:

1. Cilantro, .5 c
2. Corn kernels, 1 c
3. Vegetable broth, 2.5 c
4. Tomato paste, 6 oz.
5. Diced green chilis, 4 oz.
6. Diced tomatoes, 2 15 oz. cans
7. Salt, 1 tsp.
8. Pepper, .5 tsp.
9. Cumin, 1 tsp.
10. Chili powder, 3 T

11. Diced sweet potato
12. Diced celery, 1 c
13. Diced sweet onion, 1 c
14. Sliced carrots, 2 c
15. Dark red kidney beans, 1 can
16. Drained black beans, 2 cans

What You Do:

1. Place all of the chili ingredients, except for the cilantro, into a slow cooker.
2. Stir everything together and place the lid on the cooker and then set it to cook for six to eight hours on low.
3. Once it has finished cooking sprinkle in the cilantro. You can also top the chili with some diced avocado, sour cream, and shredded cheese.

Corn and Black Bean Salad (Dairy Free)

6 – servings

What You Need:

1. Pepper, .25 tsp.
2. Dash salt
3. Brown sugar or honey, 1 tsp.
4. Minced garlic, 1 tsp.
5. Olive oil, 2 T
6. Balsamic vinegar, .25 c
7. Minced red onion, 2 T
8. Chopped parsley, .25 c
9. Drained and rinsed black beans, 2 16 oz. cans
10. Whole kernel corn, 1 c

What You Do:

11. Place the parsley, red onion, black beans, and corn in a large bowl and mix everything together.
12. Whisk the pepper, salt, honey, garlic, lemon juice, olive oil, and balsamic vinegar together. Make sure that all of the seasonings are mixed together well.
13. Pour the dressing you just made over the corn and bean mixture.
14. Toss everything together and allow the vegetables to marinade for at least 30 minutes before you serve them.
15. This will allow all of the flavors to mix together, and the flavor will be a lot more intense.
16. Enjoy.

Spicy Peanut Vegetarian Chili (Dairy Free)

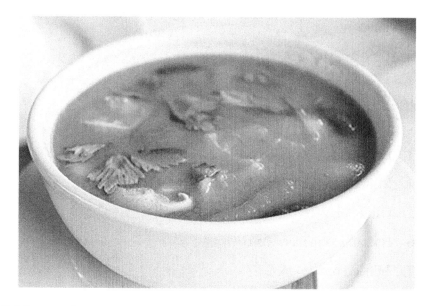

10-12 – servings

What You Need:

1. Vegetable broth, 2 c
2. Tomato sauce, 15 oz.
3. Diced tomato, 28 oz.
4. Powdered peanuts, .66 c
5. Rinsed and drained white beans, 16 oz.
6. Rinsed and drained, black beans, 16 oz.
7. Dried oregano, .25 tsp.
8. Chipotle chili pepper, 1 tsp. – optional
9. Chili powder, 2 T
10. Minced garlic, 2 cloves
11. Chopped onion, 1 c
12. Peanut oil, 1 T

What You Do:

1. Using a large Dutch oven, add in the oil and let it heat up over medium high.
2. Add in the onion and garlic and sauté them together for three to four minutes. The onions should become tender, but make sure that you don't let your garlic burn.
3. Mix in the salt, oregano, pepper, and chili powder. Allow this mixture to sauté for another two minutes, or until it becomes fragrant.
4. Mix in the broth, tomato sauce, tomatoes, powdered peanuts, corn, and cleaned beans.
5. Stir everything together and allow the mixture to come up to a boil.
6. Lower the heat down to a simmer and allow the mixture to cook for 30 minutes.
7. If you want, you can also cook this in a slow cooker.
8. Add everything to your slow cooker and mix everything together.
9. Cover your slow cooker and set it to high for two to three hours.

Black Bean, Rice, and Zucchini Skillet

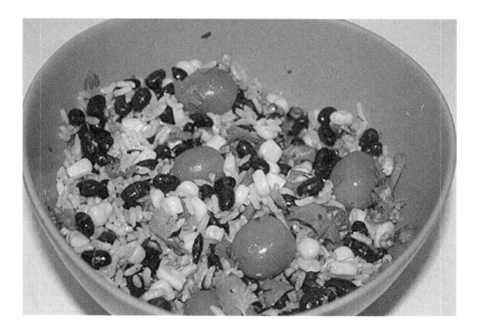

4 – servings

What You Need:

1. Monterey Jack and Cheddar cheese blend, .5 c shredded
2. Uncooked instant white rice, 1 c
3. Dried oregano, .25 tsp.
4. Water, .75 c
5. Undrained fire roasted diced tomatoes with garlic, 14.5 oz.
6. Rinsed and drained black beans, 15 oz.
7. Diced green bell pepper, .5 c
8. Chopped onion, .5 c
9. Small sliced zucchini
10. Canola oil, 1 T

What You Do:

1. Start out by heating the oil in a large pan over medium.
2. Once it is well heated, add in the bell pepper, zucchini, and onion. Allow the veggies to cook for five minutes, or until softened.
3. Make sure that you stir them occasionally.
4. Add in the oregano, water, undrained tomatoes, and beans.
5. Bring the heat up a bit and allow it to come to a boil.
6. Mix in the rice, stirring well to distribute all of the flavors.
7. Place the lid on the pan and then set it off the heat.
8. Allow the mixture to sit for seven minutes, or until the rice has absorbed all of the water.
9. Sprinkle everything with cheese and enjoy.

Seven Layer Mexican Salad

8 – servings

What You Need:

Dressing:

1. Garlic salt, .25 tsp.
2. Cumin, .5 tsp.
3. Olive oil, 1 T
4. Lime juice, 2 limes
5. Jalapeno, .5
6. Cilantro, .25 c
7. Avocado

Salad:

1. Chopped green onions, 2
2. Low-fat shredded cheddar cheese, 1 c
3. Diced tomatoes, 1 c
4. Diced bell pepper
5. Can of drained corn
6. Can of drained and rinsed black beans
7. Chopped romaine lettuce, 2 c
8. Box of Jiffy cornbread

What You Do:

1. Dressing:
2. Place all of the ingredients for the dressing in your blender and pulse them until the cilantro is well blended into the avocado and lime juice.
3. Salad:
4. First, you will need to start out by preparing the cornbread according to the directions on the box.
5. Once it has cooked through, set it aside and allow it to cool completely.
6. Once it is cooled, cut the cornbread in half and then break half of it up into little crumbs.
7. Put the crumbled cornbread into the bottom of your dish.
8. Using a trifle dish is best because you will be able to see all of the beautiful layers. You can use any bowl that you want if you don't have a trifle dish.
9. Place half of the romaine lettuce on top of the crumbled cornbread. Make sure you evenly spread it across. This is your second layer.
10. Top the lettuce with half of the black beans, making sure that they are evenly distributed.
11. Add half of the corn evenly on top of the beans.
12. Top the corn with half of the chopped bell peppers.
13. Add half of the tomatoes on top of the bell peppers, making sure that they are evenly distributed.
14. Sprinkle half of the cheddar cheese on top of the tomatoes.
15. Now drizzle on half of the salad dressing that you made earlier.

16. Repeat this process staring with the lettuce through the dressing.
17. To finish the recipe, top everything with the green onions and enjoy.
18. You can reserve the rest of the cornbread for another meal, or you can make another salad. The choice is yours.

Soft Foods

Scrambled Eggs with Black Bean Puree

1 – servings

What You Need:

Black Bean Pure:

1. Unflavored whey protein powder, 1 T
2. Vegetable or chicken broth, 2 T
3. Green enchilada sauce, 3 T
4. Rinsed black beans, .5 c

Egg:

1. Pepper, pinch
2. Salt, pinch
3. Egg

What You Do:

1. Black Bean Puree:
2. After you have rinsed off your black beans, add them to a small pot and let them heat over medium.

3. Add in two and a half T of the enchilada sauce to your beans and stir them together. Allow the mixture to cook for another two minutes.
4. Mix in the chicken broth.
5. Add the black bean mixture to your blender and mix it until completely smooth.
6. Make sure you are careful because the mixture is hot.
7. If you have an immersion blender you can use that as well to puree the beans.
8. Pour the pureed beans into a bowl.
9. Allow the pureed beans to cool slightly and then mix in the protein powder until well combined.
10. Cover them to keep them warm until you have cooked your egg.
11. Refrigerate whatever you have left over.
12. Egg:
13. Heat a pan on medium high, and as it is warming, whisk the egg together with the pepper and salt until it is well incorporated.
14. Pour the mixed egg into the hot pan. With a rubber spatula, slowly scramble the eggs until it has cooked all the way through.
15. Once the egg is nearly cooked, but it still has a liquid texture, fold it onto itself and then place it on a plate.
16. Top you egg with a T of your black bean puree you made earlier and then pour the remaining green enchilada sauce on top.

Black Bean and Lime Puree

1– servings

What You Need:

1. Unflavored protein powder, 1 T
2. Vegetable or chicken broth, .25 c
3. Jarred jalapeno juice, .5 T
4. Lime juice, .5 T
5. Rinsed black beans, .25 c

What You Do:

1. After you have rinsed your black beans, place them into a small pot and allow them to heat over medium.
2. Mix in the juice from the jalapenos and the lime juice. Stir everything together and allow it to heat through.
3. Once heated, mix in the chicken broth.
4. Pour the mixture into the blender and mix until it is completely smooth. Be careful because the mixture is hot, and make sure that you hold the lid.
5. If you have an immersion blender, you can use that as well. Pour the mixture into a bowl.
6. Allow the mixture to cool slightly and then mix in the protein powder until it is well mixed.
7. Enjoy.

Pureed Salsa and Beans

4 – servings

What You Need:

1. Unflavored whey protein powder, 1 scoop
2. Chicken broth, 2 T
3. Salsa of choice, 2 T
4. Pinto beans, 15 oz.

What You Do:

1. Place all of the ingredients into a small pot and allow it to heat up over medium high.
2. Make sure you stir it occasionally until everything has warmed through.
3. Pour the mixture into a blender.
4. Puree the mixture for a few minutes until it becomes completely smooth. Be careful because the mixture will be hot.
5. Transfer the pureed food to a serving dish.
6. Divide your leftovers into single serving containers for easier consumption later.

Egg-Chillida (Low Carb)

1 – servings

What You Need:

1. Fat-free Greek yogurt, 2 T
2. Shredded Mexican blend cheese, 1 T
3. Salsa, 2 T
4. Tofu, 1 oz.
5. Salt
6. Pepper
7. Egg white
8. Egg

What You Do:

1. Beat both the whole egg and the egg white together in a small bowl.
2. Add some nonstick spray to a pan and allow it to get heated over medium. Add the beaten egg to the heated pan, and let it spread out into a circular shape.
3. Let the egg cook on its own for a minute or so until the edges have set up. Sprinkle the top with a bit of salt and pepper as it is cooking.
4. Ease a spatula under the egg and then flip it over. There will probably be some egg that pours off, but it's not a big deal.
5. Allow the other side of the egg to cook for another minute or so, or until it has cooked all the way through.
6. Down the center of the egg, place the crumbled tofu and cheese. Roll the up like a tortilla to form your egg-chilaca. Add the yogurt and salsa on top.

Fat-Free Polenta

8 – servings

What You Need:

1. Chicken broth, 1 c
2. Fat-free milk, 2 c
3. Corn meal, 1 c

What You Do:

1. Add the broth and the milk to a medium sized pot and allow them to come up to a boil.
2. Make sure you stir the mixture constantly.
3. Once it has reached a gentle boil, whisk in the cornmeal.
4. Continue to stir the mixture for another five minutes.
5. Set the mixture off the heat and spread it into an eight by eight casserole dish or a loaf pan.
6. If you would prefer for your polenta to be soft, cover it now and allow it to chill.
7. If you would like to firm up your polenta, slide it into a 350 degree oven and allow it to bake for 14 minutes.
8. Once cooked, allow it to cool and then slice it into servings.

Conclusion

Thank for making it through to the end of *Gastric Sleeve Cookbook*, let's hope it was informative and able to provide you with all of the tools you need to achieve your goals whatever they may be.

The next step is to start enjoying these recipes. Undergoing weight loss surgery is a big step and a hard decision but deciding what to eat shouldn't have to be. Mexican dishes are delicious, and you can still enjoy them even after surgery, so start cooking today.

Finally, if you found this book useful in any way, a review on Amazon is always appreciated!

Made in the USA
Monee, IL
25 July 2020